Home Doctor:

Natural Homemade Remedies To Stay Healthy Without Pills

Table of Contents

Introduction

Congratulations! You're on your way to learning how to take control of your health by making home remedies. This book is packed with herbs, cooking ingredients, and other items you can use to help you:

- Make first aid remedies,

- Make fever reducers,

- Make tooth remedies,

- Make your own herbal baths, and

- Make your own herbal oil for massage.

This book is designed to walk you through the whole process and educate you along the way by explaining why you're using certain items and how to use those items more effectively. This will book also show you;

- What you will need to make the remedies,

- What the herbs do you will be using,

- When not to use the herbs to avoid interactions,

- How to store them, and

- How long they last,

By the time you have read through the following chapters, you will find yourself wondering what else you can do with the herbs and things you find around your home. Let's get started!

Chapter 1 – Getting Started

Every new thing you learn needs the proper tools to do it right. Don't worry. When making home remedies, it is best to avoid contamination as much as possible, but it won't require you turning your kitchen into a laboratory, and most of the things on the following list are probably already in your home:

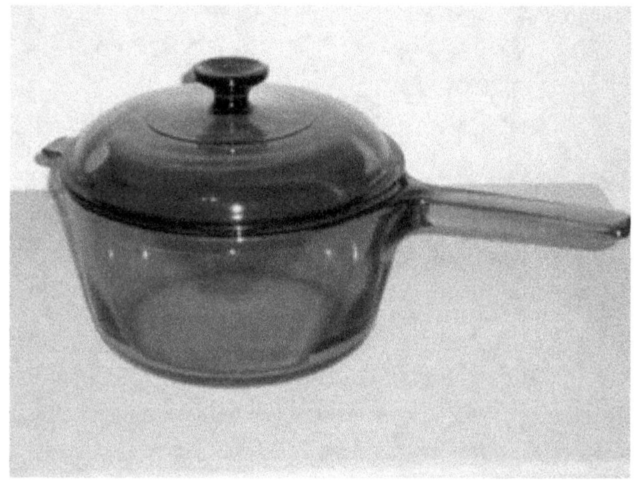

•Glass or porcelain pot or tea pot

- o Water can leach the properties of the metals it is boiled in. This can make the remedy have an unintended taste or not work as well.

- o Vision cookware is best, but you can still find porcelain tea pots on sale in department stores, if you don't already have the pots.

- Wooden spoons and ladles

- Coffee filters or cheesecloth

    o Some remedies require you to strain the herbs from the tea. These are two highly recommended ways of doing it.

- Porcelain or glass cups

    o This is for steeping teas.

- Dark glass bottles or jars

    o The less light going through the glass when storing oils and ointments, the longer those remedies last.

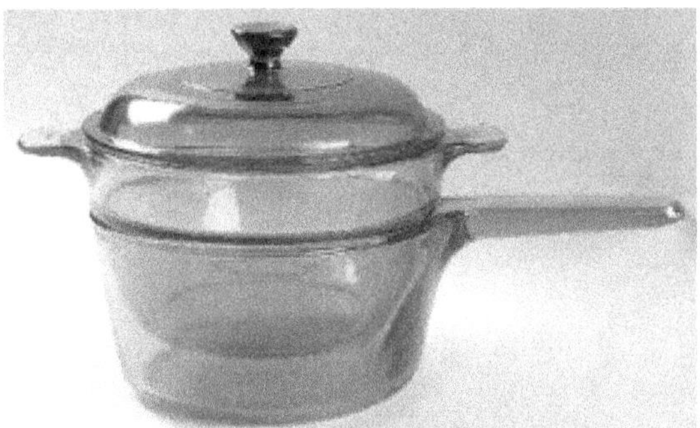

- Double boiler or Bain Marie

    o Some remedies will call for you to gently heat ingredients without them touching water. Again, please use either glass or porcelain.

- Porcelain or glass baking pan

- Crock pot

    o This is for making your herbal oils quicker than the conventional way.

- Candle Warmer

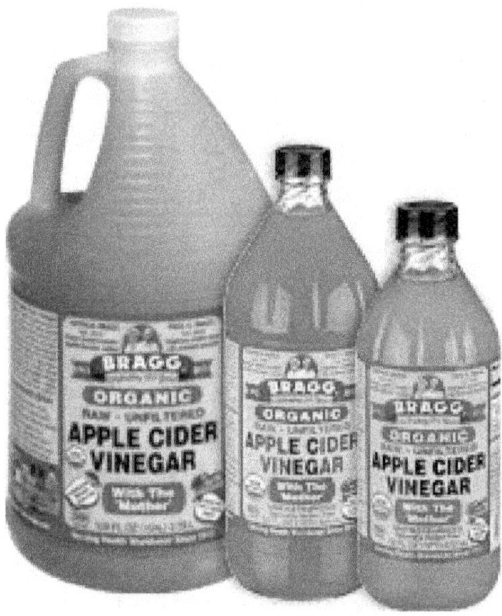

oIf you don't have an essential oil diffuser, this is the next best thing. You can place the undiluted essential oils directly on the warmer.

Here are a few things you may not have thought of that are already in your kitchen:

•Coffee grinds

oThese are perfect for facial masks and scrubs.

•Brown Sugar

oFor sugar scrubs

- Baking soda

    o   For bath salts

- Sea salt

    o   For salt scrubs and bath salts

- Epsom Salts

    o   For mineral baths

- Borax

    o   This is a natural mineral that boosts that action of mineral bath salts.

- Whole Oats

- Ground and added in place of salt, it makes for a soothing mineral bath.

- Vinegar

    - Apple Cider Vinegar with the mother.

    - This is wonderful when mixed with a tea for cleansing the skin, and removing build-up from hair products.

- Olive Oil

    - Great for herbal oils

- Coconut Oil

- - Just like Olive oil, but it has more healing properties and you can even make it into ointments.

- Eggs

    - Good for conditioning hair.

    - Good for the skin as well.

As you can see, there are a lot of things you already have you can use to make remedies without breaking the bank. I will probably mention more that are not the list above in the recipes as we go on.

Chapter 2 – Your Spice Rack

You use it every day to add flair and flavor to your dishes. A little oregano here and a pinch of basil there, and you can even turn left-overs into a whole new dish, but did you know many of the herbs you cook with can also help heal you as well?

Allspice

This wonderful little herb who lends its flavor to many island dishes, also helps in cases of indigestion, intestinal cramping, and eve help relieve the swelling and of swollen joints from arthritis. It can be made into a tea, into an oil and even a bath.

Basil

This herb, which is in many households, is a champ when it comes to remedies which are home-made. It helps to tame gas, soothes nerves, calms nausea, can be used as an antihistamine, and is a good disinfectant. You can make it into a tea or oil.

Cinnamon

Cinnamon is used in confections and island dishes. The essential oil of this herb is used to calm the nerves and a nervous stomach. The powdered cinnamon is no different. It also provides natural caffeine, just a little bit. This herb is great as an oil.

Cayenne

Famous for adding heat to chili, Cayenne is also helpful in cases of intestinal problems, indigestion, and can loosen up phlegm caused by congestion. great for poultices, capsules, and ointments.

Cloves

This is another good one for indigestion and nausea. The juice from a single clove can stop nausea and the convulsion related to it. Just chew it to get the juice and spit out the clove.

Garlic

This wonder herb is known to boost the immune system, help lower high blood pressure and cholesterol, and even help in cases of congestion. You can eat it straight, but it's better served as an oil.

Ginger

Chewing on this herb in its candied form can help allay motion sickness. It is also great for lessening the severity and duration of colds and flu. The fresh juice is good in poultices and teas.

Bay (laurel) Leaves

We add these to stews and sometimes even chili, but did you know it can help heal a sprain, earaches, and even removes blockages that cause infections? It's true!

Marjoram

Another favorite in Italian dishes, Marjoram also helps to speed the healing in cases of sprains and can also heal bruises. Good in rubs and soaks.

Parsley

Yes, the green leafy spring on expensive restaurant plates is there for a reason. It helps to combat heartburn, gas, and bad breath. It can also help break-up kidney stones and treat insect bites. You can apply the juice by crushing the herb.

Pepper, Black

Usually paired with salt in restaurants, this herb, when made into a paste, can help soothe bronchitis and other chronic respiratory problems. You can put this in ointments and oils.

Onion

Though not an herb per se, can help in cases of water retention, earaches, coughs and colds. Make into an oil.

Rosemary

The herb that makes chicken sing and soups taste wonderful helps treat headaches, nervous tension, a nervous stomach, cleanse the face, and can even help to stimulate hair growth. Great in teas, oils, and soaks.

Sage

This is an herb no one that makes home remedies is caught without. It has antiseptic properties, anti-inflammation properties, can draw out toxins from bug bites, and even help to treat abscesses in the mouth. It's also helpful in healing ulcers. It's great in washes, teas, and ointments.

Thyme

This Italian herb is also known for helping in cases of sinus problems. It helps to break up impacted mucous. You can use it like Sage.

It's a long list, but a very helpful one when you're looking for something to make and have handy in case something happens or someone gets sick.

Herbs and Essential Oils you can add to it.

This list will cover essential oils and herbs you can find in health food and herb shops that are affordable. Adding these to your home remedy list will have you prepared for anything.

Aloe

The all-natural gel or juice is the best. Most of the aloes you get in bottles during the summer have been diluted with alcohol. You can use this as a base for many spot treatments.

Calendula Petals

Most commonly known as Marigold, this herb can speed clotting and is a strong antiviral in cases of colds and flu.

Chamomile
This herb can be found in the tea section of any grocery store. You can combine it with some of the cooking herbs above for skin problems and soothing the stomach.

Echinacea
Many places sell this as a tea as well, which comes in handy if you're making poultices or compresses. It boosts the immune system and speeds the healing of cuts, scrapes, and bruises.

Feverfew
Coupled with Rosemary, it's a powerful punch for treating headaches, migraines, and cluster headaches. This herb alone can do it, but sometimes even the best herb for the job can use a helping hand.

Green Tea
Though many don't consider this tea an herb, it actually is. It is packed with antioxidants and antivirals to help you take care of mouth problems and kick colds.

White Oak Bark
This one can be found in health food stores, herb shops and online. As a powder, you can make into a poultice for bug bites. It draws out the toxins.

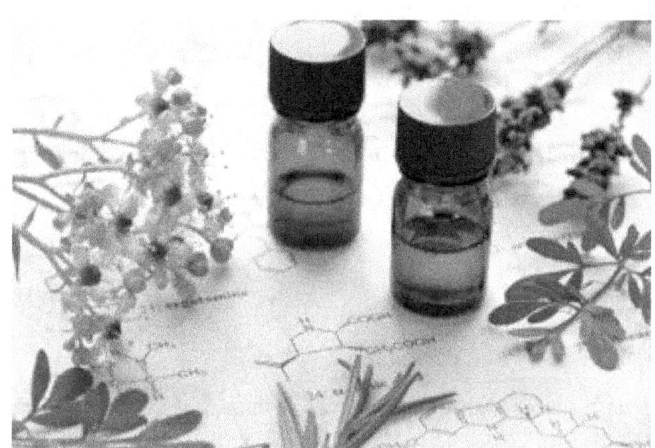

Lavender Essential oil

This versatile essential oil can help in first aid heal burns and sooth itching. It also helps to reduce inflammation.

Lemon Essential oil

This oil can kill germs and when used with Peppermint, Echinacea, and Sage, it can help to speed the healing of cuts, scrapes and bruises.

Peppermint Essential oil

This oil not only smells heavenly, but can be used in a pinch, mixed with a lotion as a penetrating chest rub or added to a poultice to help open up a congested chest. You can also add it to water to make a disinfectant and even deter fleas.

Tea Tree Essential oil

This essential oil is a great germ fighter. You can add it to water for a spot disinfectant or even put a few drops on a candle warmer to kill airborne germs.

There are a lot more herbs you can get to supplement this list, but this is a list of the most readily available and most affordable. Some herbs and essential oils can cost upwards of $20.00 or more for the smallest of bottles.

Chapter 3 – A word to the wise...

When taking herbal supplements and remedies on a regular basis, you need to take heed about possible interactions that may happen if you are on prescription medications. These can range from mildly irritating to possible life-threatening.

Blood thinners and Blood pressure medications

There are some herbs that can thin the blood, lower, and even raise blood pressure. If you are taking any of these types of prescription medicine, avoid these types of herbs.

If you are on high blood pressure medications, avoid using Rosemary in therapeutic does as it may cause a spike in blood pressure, counteracting the medication.

Antidepressants

If you are on antidepressants, avoid taking herbals that do the same thing. This will cause euphoria and can lead to injury down the road.

Diabetes

There are herbs out there that can raise or lower your blood sugar. Some of these, like Stevia and Nopal, can be fine when you monitor your blood sugar and adjust accordingly, but do so cautiously. Golden Seal, an immune booster, can drastically lower blood sugar and should be avoided by people with blood sugar problems.

Auto-immune diseases

We all want to feel better, but if you are suffering from an auto-immune disease, consult your doctor and a naturopath to see if taking herbs can be beneficial and which ones to avoid so you don't block the action of existing treatments.

You and your doctor

If you are going in for tests and you're taking herbal supplements, you may have to stop taking those as well. Many herbs, taken in either maintenance or therapeutic does, can skew test results. Let your doctor know what you are taking.

Chapter 4 – How to prepare them.

This is the part of the book you've been waiting for, but you're going to need to learn a few terms and preparations first. So, let's get that list out of the way.

Compress

This can made from teas and essential oils. This is a bowl of warm to hot water with medicinal properties which can be placed, via a clean damp towel, on the affected area. It is switched out when the towel gets cool.

Decoction

This is a teas made from boiling roots, stems, and bark. These ingredients take longer to extract the medicinal properties out of them. They need 20 minutes on a low boil. These can store in a refrigerator for about a week.

Facial Mask

This is a type of poultice you put on your face. These are usually one-shot treatments.

Herbal Baths

This is the practice of taking four ounces of herbs and sewing, or placing them, into a pillow case or other bag that allow the water to flow into it. You place it in a tub of warm to hot running water and soak up the medicine. These are one-shot.

Herbal oil

You can make this two ways:

1. Adding an ounce of dried herbs to a pint of oil in a glass jar and leaving it for three weeks in a warm place.

2. Adding an ounce of dried herbs to a pint of oil in a crock pot on low overnight.

I personally use the second method. Crock pots get just hot enough to help release the heating properties of the herbs without frying the plant material.

Depending on the oil you use and how you store it, an herbal oil can last up to six months in a cool dry place.

Infusion

This is a tea made from the leaves and flowers of the herbs. Traditionally, you make it buy running a pint of water through herbs placed on a strainer, but for book purposes, you can make them buy adding water to a cup or bowl which has the herbs already in them. These take 10 minutes to steep to get the most benefit from the medicinal properties. These last about as long as decoctions.

Lotions

More often than not, you will be using unscented lotion you can find at any store. You can add small amounts of herbs and essential oil to this for healing purposes. These are one-shot as you make it as you need it.

Massage oils

This is an oil to which herbs or essential oils or both have been added. You can use this to sooth tight muscles, treat bruises, and even soften skin, depending on the ingredients. These can last about as long as herbal oils.

Mineral Baths

This is a combination of Borax, Sea Salt, Epsom Salt, and Baking Soda. You can add herbs and essential oils to the mix to speed healing, detox your body, or just relax. If you have high blood pressure, it is recommended you substitute the salts for ground oatmeal. If you make a large batch, it can store up to six months before the potency starts to wane.

Mouthwash

These can be made by using existing mouthwash, vodka, or another clear alcohol. If you do not drink, you can use witch hazel.

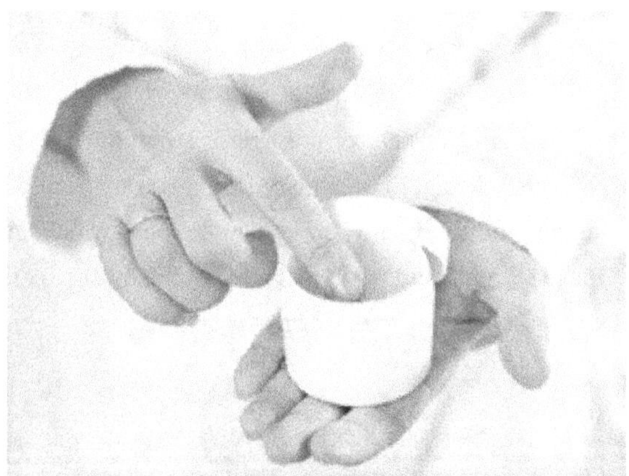

Ointments

These can be tricky to make, but they can last a while. You start by warming a base oil and adding the herbs. You then strain out the herbs and add the oil to a double boiler. You then add beeswax to the oil. If you are adding essential oils to this, it is recommended you wait unit the mixture is Luke warm.

Poultice

I've mentioned this one a couple of times already. A poultice is a thick paste made of herbs, essential oils, and water. This can be applied directly to wounds and bruises to pull out infections and speed healing. These are generally one-shot as you make them when you need them.

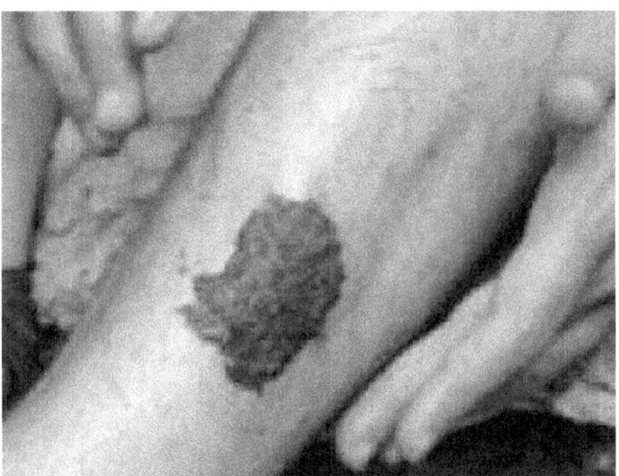

Syrups

These are cough syrups you can make at home with water, herbs, and honey. It takes two ounces of the herb, one quart of water, and two ounces of honey. These can last up to a week in the refrigerator.

Wound wash

Just as it sounds, you mix tea and essential oils in a squeeze bottle and squirt it in the scrape or cut to wash out any dirt particles and clean the wound. This is a quick way to clean and disinfect a cut or scrape. These are immediate use.

Chapter 5 – The Remedies

Now we're ready to get to it. These recipes will start with the top of the body and their way down.

Headache Remedies
Rosemary and Thyme Sinus Pack
1 tbsp ground whole oats

1 tsp Rosemary leaves

1 tsp Thyme leaves

1/4 boiled water

5 Drops Peppermint essential oil

2 Drops of Lavender essential oi

2 Drops of Lemon essential oil

- Add the Rosemary and Thyme to the boiled water.

- Cover and let steep for ten minutes

- Add just enough of the strong infusion to make a paste.

- Add the essential oils and mix well.

- Place the poultice around the eyes, being careful not get any in the eyes.

- Leave on for twenty minutes before washing off.

Headache Tea

1 tsp Feverfew

1/2 tsp Rosemary

1 Drop Peppermint essential oil

- Boil one cup of water, about 6 ounces.

- Add the water the herbs and let steep for ten minutes.

- Strain out the herbs, add the peppermint, and a little honey.

Headache Herbal oil

1/2 Ounce of Feverfew

1/2 Ounce of Rosemary

1 pint of Olive oil

1/2 tbsp of peppermint

- Place the herbs in a crock pot.

- Add the oil

- Let run on low overnight.

- Add the essential oil.

- Mix well.

- Apply to temples, base of the neck, and the bridge of your nose.

Fevers

For a head cold I

Compress

2 Tbsp Echinacea

1/2 tbsp Rosemary

1/2 tbsp Thyme

1/2 tbsp Feverfew

- Boil water and add the above ingredients.

- Strain out the herbs

- Damp a clean cloth

- Place on forehead

- change when the cloth is cool

- If needed, reheat the water.

Flu Compress

3 Cups water

25 Drops Lavender Essential oil

25 Drops Peppermint essential oil

2 tbsp Thyme

2 tbsp Feverfew

- Boil the herbs in the water

- Add the essential oils

- Damp a clean cloth

- Place cloth on forehead

- Replace cloth when cool.

Your Mouth

When your mouth is healthy, your body can stave off a lot of infections. When you don't take proper care of your teeth and gums, you can run into problems.

Abscess Wash

1 Cup of Listerine or other unflavored antiseptic mouthwash.

2 Tablespoons Sage

1 tablespoon Echinacea

1 Tablespoon White Oak Bark

35 Drops of Tea Tree oil

- Place all of the ingredients in a jar with a tight lid.

- Shake and place in a dark, cool, place.

- Shake once in the morning and once at night.

- Do this for three days.

- Strain the herbs out.

- Use the normal amount of mouthwash before brushing your teeth.

The Oak Bark and the Sage will pull out the infection. The Tea Tree and Echinacea will kill it. The Sage will also bring down the swelling.

Gingivitis Rub

1/2 Cup of Coconut oil

2 tbsp Sage

1 tbsp Echinacea or Green Tea

10 Drops of Peppermint Essential oil

15 Drops of Lavender Essential oil

- Heat the herbs in the oil overnight in a crock pot

- Using a cheesecloth, strain out the herbs.

- Place the oil in a dark glass container.

- Add the essential oils when the oil is Luke Warm

- Apply to the gums after you have brushed your teeth.

The herbs and essential oils will work together to help bring down swelling and repair the damage to your gums while preventing infections.

Chest congestion

We all get those chest colds. We feel like we can't draw a breath without coughing. Coughing is the body's natural way of getting rid of viruses and infections. It may be gross to think about, but when you cough something up, don't swallow it. Spit it out. It will speed your recovery.

Chest pack

1 Cup hot water

1/2 Fresh Ginger root crushed

2 tbsp Cinnamon

15 Drops Peppermint Essential oil

15 Drops of Lemon Essential oil

- Crush the fresh Ginger in a bowl to retain the juice

- Add the Cinnamon

- Add the Essential oils

- Add just enough of the water to make the paste warm.

- Apply the paste to the chest and cover with plastic wrap.

- When it is completely cool, remove and shower as normal.

Cold and Flu Tea

1 pot of water (12 cups)

1 tbsp of Echinacea

1/2 tbsp Ginger

1 tbsp Thyme

1 tbsp Feverfew

1 tbsp Calendula petals

1/2 tbsp Chamomile

- Mix all of the herbs in the coffee filter.

* Brew a pot as normal.

* Sweeten with raw honey

* Add Lemon Juice

* You can also add 5 drops of peppermint essential oil, but that is optional.

Chest Ointment

1/4 Cup of Cayenne Pepper

1/4 cup of fresh Ginger

1/2 cup of Echinacea

1 Cup of Olive oil

1/4 Cup beeswax

25 Drops of Peppermint Essential oil

20 Drops of Lavender Essential oil

10 drops of Tea Tree essential oil

Dark glass jars to store it in

* Place the herbs and oil in a crock pot overnight.

* Use a cheese cloth to strain it out.

* Put the oil back in the double boiler and heat

* Add the beeswax and wait until it melts

* Pour into your containers

* Mix the essential oils

- Add the essential oils when the main mixture is warm and not hot.

- Apply to the chest and under nose as needed to break up sinus and chest pressure.

Cold and Flu Bath

1/4 Cup Fine Sea Salt

1/4 Cup Epsom Salt

1/4 Cup Baking Soda

1/8 Cup Borax

3 tbsp ground fresh ginger

2 tbsp Rosemary leaves, ground

3 tbsp ground Echinacea

1/4 Cup Olive oil

10 Drops Peppermint

10 Drops Lavender Essential oil

5 Drops Tea Tree oil

- Add all the dry ingredients first.

- Mix all the oils separately

- Slowly add the oil to the dry ingredients.

- Mix well and place in an air-tight container

- Leave it sit overnight.

- Add 1/4 Cup to running water

Burns

You can put a few drops of the Lavender Essential oil on the burn, but constantly applying it neat (not diluted) can cause dermatitis. It is best to mix 6 drops of the essential oil with a tablespoon of olive oil.

You can also use this ointment:

Burn ointment

1/2 Cup Olive oil

1/4 cup Beeswax

1/4 Cup Calendula petals

25 Drops of Lavender essential oil

- Place the oil and herb in a crock pot overnight

- Use a cheesecloth to strain out the herb

- Reheat the oil in a double boiler

- Melt the beeswax

- Add the mixture to a jar with a tight lid.

- Wait until it is Luke Warm to add the Lavender

- Use on the burn area

Quick fix burn treatment

1 tbsp Aloe gel

6 drops Lavender essential oil

- Mix and apply to burn area

Wound wash

Let's face it. If you have kids, you're going to need a better, and faster way, to clean out a cut or scrape when they come home battered from a day outside or at the park. They're kids, and they play hard.

4 Ounces of warm water

25 Drops of Peppermint Essential oil

25 Drops of Tea Tree Essential oil

4-ounce squirt bottle

- Place all the ingredients in the bottle and shake vigorously
- Squirt into the wound

That's it. It will not only wash the dirt of, or out, it will also disinfect the wound.

Bruise ointment

1/2 Cup of Olive oil

1/4 Beeswax

1/4 Cup Marjoram

1/4 Cup Echinacea

- Steep the herbs overnight in a crock pot on low.

- Use a cheesecloth to strain them out.

- Reheat the oil in a double boiler

- Melt the Beeswax

- Add the ointment to dark glass jars.

- Wait until it cools.

- Apply to bruises.

First aid ointment

1 Cup of Olive oil

1/2 Cup of Beeswax

1/4 Cup of Sage

4 Large Bay leaves

1/4 Cup of Marjoram

1/4 Cup of Calendula Petals

1/4 Cup of Echinacea

20 Drops of Lavender Essential oil

20 Drops of Peppermint Essential oil

10 Drops of Tea Tree Oil

- Steep the herbs overnight in a crock pot on low

- Using a cheesecloth, strain out the herbs

- Place the oil in a double boiler

- Melt the beeswax into the olive oil

- Mix the essential oils.

- Place the ointment into dark glass jars.

- When it is Luke Warm, add equal amounts of the essential oil blend

- Apply to cuts, scrapes, bruises or other wounds.

- You can even apply it to bandage and then the wound.

Herbal bath for sprains

Depending on whether it's your back or a smaller part of the body, you will need to scale it appropriately.

1 ounce of Marjoram

1 ounce of Bay leaves

Reusable filter bag

- Place the herbs in the bag

- Place the bag in a tub of running hot water

- Swirl the water around before laying the tub.

- Soak the sprained body part.

- you can scale it down to coffee pot size by doing the following:

  - 3 coffee scoops of Marjoram

- 4 bay leaves

- Brew like it's coffee

- Add to a foot soak for feet, elbows or ankles.

Mineral Foot Soak

Achy feet need love, too. They carry us hither and yon without a complaint, most of the time.

1/4 Cup Sea salt, fine

1/4 Cup Epsom Salt

1/4 cup baking soda

1/8 cup Olive oil

1/8 cup Ground sage

10 Drops Peppermint Oil

10 Drops Lavender oil

- Mix all the dry ingredient and set them aside

- Mix all the oils well

- Slowly add the oils to the dry ingredients

- Place in an air-tight container overnight.

- Add 1/8 cup to warm water in a foot soak/massager.

Tight and achy muscle rub

After a long day of stooping, lifting, and moving around, your back may feel tight, strained and even hurt. A good massage oil will do the trick.

Word to the wise: Do NOT massage pulled muscles. You will make them worse.

1 Cup Olive oil

1/4 cup Black Pepper

1/4 cup sage

1/4 Cup Allspice

1/4 Echinacea

25 Drops of Lavender essential oil

25 Drops of Peppermint

- Steep the herbs in the oil in a crock pot overnight

- Strain out the herbs

- Wait until the oil cools to add the essential oils

- Mix well

- Massage into the tight muscles.

- You can even add this to the base mineral bath mixture above for a nice relaxing bath.

- You can even make this mixture into an ointment to rub into smaller areas like knees and elbows.

Quick and dirty remedies

- 1 tsp of Baking soda in a 1/4 cup of warm water can alleviate a case of heartburn.

- Adding three drops of peppermint essential oil to a cotton ball and placing it on a heating vent in your car can ease you tension on the ride home.

- Putting 50 drops of Lemon essential oil in your rinse water can sanitize surfaces as you clean.

- Making onion oil and putting a few drops in your ear can alleviate an ear ache.

- One teaspoon of Apple Cider Vinegar in a 1/4 cup of warm water can dry up weeping eczema and psoriasis.

- Putting used Green Tea bags on your eyes can help with wrinkles and bags around the eye area.

- Making cucumber oil from the skin can tighten skin and help clear up acne.

- Cucumber juice added to Witch Hazel is a great base for a facial astringent.

- Adding two drops of Lavender Essential oil to your baby's soap relaxes them and helps them sleep.

- Adding six drops of Lavender essential oil to a candle warmer in a baby's room can help them sleep soundly.

- Adding ten drops of Lavender essential oil to a candle warmer in an adult's room can allay anxiety and help you fall asleep faster.

- Adding 1/4 tsp of Tea tree oil to a bowl of warm water can kill fleas when you dunk a flea comb in it.

- Making a tea with cloves and placing it in a spray bottle can be an effective bug repellant. Spray it on lawn furniture and even on your pets.

- Adding Peppermint essential oil to baking soda can kill fleas in the carpet. Just mix 10 drops per two tablespoons of baking soda. Wait until it's dry before you sprinkle in your carpet. Work it into your carpet, and then vacuum it up. You can use 5 drops of Tea Tree and Five drops of Peppermint essential oils for a double punch.

Conclusion

Natural health and home remedies go hand-in-hand. From what your grandmother taught you mother and was passed on to you and what you have picked up in your life, there is a way to treat cuts, scrapes and achy muscles without a trip to the doctor and spending budget breaking dollars on prescription medications.

The basic information is the book is in hopes to get you started on a healthier life and a way to apply first aid and take care of everyday aches. It's not intended to diagnose or treat serious illnesses. In the case of such illnesses or severe injuries, please consult a licensed physician.

If you are looking for more information, keep an eye out for future books. You can also join groups and forums online to further your curiosity. Online communities can steer you making more home remedies and where to find the ingredients without breaking the bank.

May you live a long and healthy life.

FREE Bonus Reminder

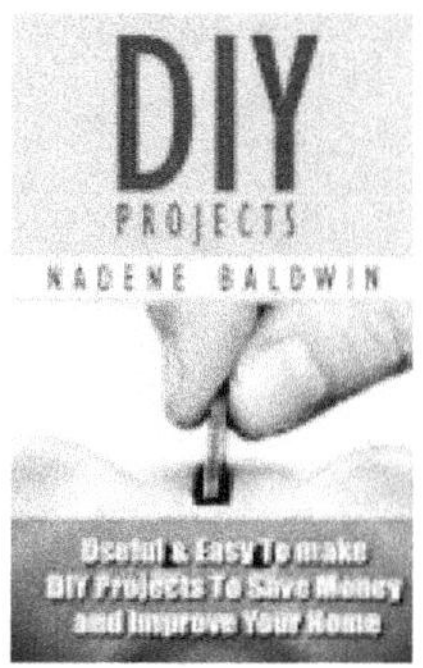

If you have not grabbed it yet, please go ahead and download your special bonus report *"DIY Projects. 13 Useful & Easy To Make DIY Projects To Save Money & Improve Your Home!"*

Simply Click the Button Below

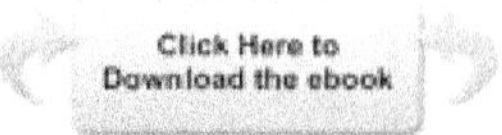

OR **Go to This Page**

http://diyhomecraft.com/free

BONUS #2: More Free & Discounted Books or Products

Do you want to receive more Free/Discounted Books or Products?

We have a mailing list where we send out our new Books or Products when they go free or with a discount on Amazon. Click on the link below to sign up for Free & Discount Book & Product Promotions.

=> Sign Up for Free & Discount Book & Product Promotions <=

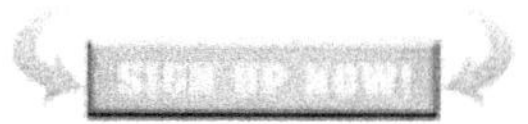

OR Go to this URL

http://zbit.ly/1WBb1Ek

www.ingramcontent.com/pod-product-compliance
Lightning Source LLC
Chambersburg PA
CBHW050708250726
48662CB00002B/916